SWEET SURRENDER

How to Become Your Own Best Health Advocate

By

Kristi Jacques Falk

CONTENTS

DEDICATION

I dedicate this book first of all, to my parents. To my father, John Hubert Jacques, for being such an inspiration and hero to me. He truly was the greatest man I have ever known. To my mother, Carol Hutto Jacques for her love, dedication and her constant search for better ways of living with diabetes. She continues to teach me so much. I love you!

I also dedicate this to my husband, Dr. Daniel Falk, who has been my biggest supporter. He has always been by my side nudging me gently, but boldly in the right direction.

Lastly, this book is for anyone who may be struggling with an illness without knowing what to do. I'd like my story to be an inspiration to you on your journey. No matter how frustrated you feel, don't give up and don't stop trying. Most importantly, remember that you are not alone.

INTRODUCTION

I wrote this book because, as someone who has spent a lifetime dealing with type-1 diabetes and DIY-ing my health care to overcome many health struggles, I wanted my story to give people hope that things can get better. I know how frustrating it can be to feel awful and not find any answers from the medical community. But I also know persistence in advocating for yourself pays off.

Now, as the director of the Diabetes Wellness Council, a non-profit located in South Carolina that focuses on Diabetes prevention and education, I work with many who simply don't know how to advocate for their own health. Too many Americans suffering from the effects of chronic illness or pain do whatever the doctor tells them, without giving it a second thought. It's time for this to change!

So, this book isn't really about me. It's about YOU. I want you to know that it is absolutely okay to question your doctor and get a second, or even a third, opinion. With the information available to all of us at the touch of a button, we are no longer at the mercy of a few experts convinced that what works for one patient must work for every other patient. Please don't misunderstand my intention here. I'm by no means suggesting you try every crackpot remedy you read about online promising a cure. Rather, I'm suggesting you read widely, keep an open mind, think things through for yourself, and bring questions to medical professionals.

It is also my intention to empower you to speak up, ask questions, look things up, and even work in partnership with your doctor to come up with solutions to your health care concerns. There is simply no better person to gauge what is going on inside your own body, than you.

Finally, I want you to know in reading my story that you are not alone in your health struggles. There is a lot that even the most intelligent medical minds have yet to figure out about human health and disease. But if we accept that someone in a whitecoat has all the answers, then we are not participating in our own wellness. We are giving over our power to others.

This book is not meant to be medical advice or to replace your doctor. It is simply meant to tell my story of becoming my own best health advocate and offer you a bridge to become your own best health advocate. What could be a more hopeful message?

CHAPTER 1:
FROM ANGST TO ACCEPTANCE

It was February 1983. I was 12 ½ years old and I was sick. I had been sick for awhile, according to my mother, and was getting sicker by the day. I was always thirsty, going to the bathroom often, and throwing up frequently. She sensed something was really wrong and took me to see our family doctor. He ran some blood work. He told me that he was testing me for diabetes on the request of my mother. I was angry. Very angry. The only experience I had ever had with diabetes was our nextdoor neighbor, we will call him Mr. W. He was severely overweight and in a wheelchair, due to the fact that both of his legs had been amputated because of diabetes. How could my mother think that I had something like that? I was very angry.

The next day, I was feeling even worse and was taken to the hospital. I remember being carried to the car because I could barely move. I also remember being wheeled around on a gurney in the emergency room when the doctor there asked me how long I had been diabetic. That was how I found out. My mother had been right. Of course now, I am truly grateful that she knew the warning signs then, otherwise, I may not even be here today.

Now I know that the reason I felt so badly the first time I was hospitalized for diabetes was because I was going into ketoacidosis a life-threatening condition where the blood sugar has been too high for too long. This is where I was at the time. I had been losing weight, I was thirsty all of the time, always going to the bathroom, vomiting and have severe lethargy. My blood sugar was extremely high and I was admitted to the hospital. I could barely move; I really didn't know what was really going on. I was almost comatose. I was in the hospital for about two weeks.

Two weeks is a long time to be in the hospital, especially for a 12-year-old girl just finding out that she was diagnosed with diabetes. The short story about why I was there for so long, is because, quite simply, I am stubborn. It would turn out later that being stubborn would serve me well in living with diabetes. But at this particular time in my life, my stubbornness just meant a lot of long, boring days and nights in a hospital bed. I was not accepting of my condition and refused to learn how to give myself insulin injections. I wanted absolutely no part of it. The nurses were patient and brought me orange after orange to practice on but it didn't help. Sticking an orange is easy enough, but there was NO way I was sticking a needle anywhere on my own body. NO way.

Then finally one day, my doctor came in the room with a syringe and a bottle of saline. He rolled up his sleeve and said that I could practice on him. Well, that seemed like a great idea! It felt better than punching him would (or so I imagined, because sometimes I did want to punch him). So I did it and eventually gave in to trying it on myself. They let me go home after that.

So let me tell you a little about my parents. I owe them everything. I wouldn't be here without them of course, but they also made me who I am today. They were very patient with me in the beginning. They were concerned of course and only wanted the best for me.

My father was quite simply the best man I have ever known. He was kind, generous, loving, selfless, hard working, forgiving, funny and just an all around wonderful man. He was outgoing and everybody was his friend. If he really liked you, you were "adopted" into our family forever. I loved that about him. I try to be as outgoing as him but it doesn't always work. I am a bit quieter and more reserved. But I work on it all of the time. He was also extremely passionate about the causes he cared about. When I was diagnosed with Type 1 diabetes, he joined the local chapter of the Juvenile Diabetes Foundation, which later became the Juvenile Diabetes Research Foundation. He wanted to find out everything he could, find support from other parents and he really wanted to find a cure for me. I remember just watching him at some of the meetings and talking to people. His face would just light up and he always showed up with a big smile. He won people over immediately and I was always so proud that he was my dad. He quickly became the president of the chapter. He was a born leader and everyone loved him and was eager to follow. He went to Washington D.C. on many occasions, lobbying for more research dollars to find a cure. So I believe that I get that passion from him. The passion for helping others, for doing better and doing more. I would love nothing more than an actual cure for this disease.

My mother is amazing. She is intelligent, strong and loving. She taught me an extremely important lesson about health. When I was young, she made me eat my vegetables. Even just a little. If I didn't like it, too bad. I had to at least eat a bite or two each time. I used to despise broccoli and Brussel sprouts. Now they are among my favorite vegetables, simply because I had to try it every time. I thank her for that. She also taught me to ask questions. To look things up, do my own research.

When I was first diagnosed, my doctor at the time told me that I would need to "eat healthy", eat a "diabetic diet" from then on. He didn't say anything specific. Just eat healthy. No direction. That was it. So my mother went to work looking things up, trying new recipes (some worked, some did not). If she had a new recipe for a casserole on the table, my father would look at me with a terrified look on his face. We never knew exactly what to expect from her experiments, but most of it was delicious. There was always a running family joke about her "burn and serve rolls." She was striving to do her best for me and my health. I think that every parent wants their child to be as healthy as possible. At least I hope that's true. My mother definitely did and does. I can't thank her enough for everything she taught me.

To us, eating healthier meant eating vegetables. I lived in a small South Carolina town called Norway until I was five. We had a big garden, grape vines and lots of open land to play in. Eating vegetables wasn't really an issue for me since I had always eaten my veggies. When I was little, I had to at least taste a vegetable I didn't like or didn't know, every time it was on my plate. So I am truly thankful that I was required to "taste" everything every time. I see so many kids in some of my programs who eat few vegetables simply because they don't like them and the parents don't want to argue. I've seen it time and time again, even in my own family. I will argue however, that proper nutrition should start at a very early age. The sooner you get your kids tasting different vegetables, the more likely it is that they will be a little healthier in adulthood. Good nutrition is important at any age, but especially in the formative years.

Like I said, we had to do our own research and figure out what it meant to eat healthy and live healthy as a diabetic. At this time, there were no home glucometers, which are small handheld machines that use a drop of blood to find out your blood sugar level. What I used were urine sticks to see if my blood sugar was so high that it was spilling into my urine. The strips tested for ketones in the urine which meant extremely high blood sugar. Too high of a reading created the possibility of going into ketoacidosis, like I did when first diagnosed. That is not something I wanted to experience again, so I tried to stay on top of it. I tried to do everything I was supposed to, taking my insulin, eating "healthy" and getting some exercise. Of course, I didn't always succeed. Sometimes it tested positive for high sugar, but I think most of the time it was pretty good.

I did pretty well for the most part. There were times when I would get angry and would act out. I remember eating an entire snickers bar in front of my parents just to hurt them for "doing this to me." I remember standing there in front of my mother with a scowl on my face, opening the wrapper and eating the entire candy bar right in front of her then shouting, "I HOPE You're happy!" I absolutely regret that, but I was a kid and was hurt, scared and confused. Like I said before, I was really stubborn and in my pre-teen years, so I was even more difficult. I know now that perhaps my blood sugar was out of range, either high or low, to cause such behavior. Testing then was only through the urine strip, so I had no way of knowing for sure. Things are so much easier and faster today. For today's youth going through this kind of diagnosis, remember that it really is easier now. It's easier to keep track of your blood sugar all of the time. I really wish I had that kind of technology when I was first diagnosed.

My parents, knowing how I felt, started sneaking out to go to the JDF meetings. They knew I still really had not accepted it and wanted no part of it. Not only that, but I felt alone and so very different from everyone at school that I didn't want to run into any other kids my age that might be there. One day a stranger knocked on the door. I said no thank you, closed the door and told my parents it was a Jehovah's witness. It was of course, the president of the local JDF chapter. My bad.

When they explained to me who he was and that he had a son close to my age that also had diabetes, just like me, I decided to take a leap of faith. I started going to the meetings and meeting other kids like me. Diabetics. Normal. Active. I started to feel better and not so alone. We quickly became an integral part of the organization and worked so hard to raise money and awareness. I started to question things and learn how to take better care of myself. At a very young age, I wrote for a local newspaper in an interview I did with a family with a diabetic toddler. I even took pictures. I believe I still have a copy of that article. In middle school I had to write a research paper. So I interviewed an actual medical researcher at The Medical University of South Carolina about his job. I wanted to learn everything, and I thought maybe that was something I would be interested in pursuing later in life.

So I continued to eat my veggies, I took PE class in school, tried dance and gymnastics (neither of which I was very good at), and I did everything a normal kid would do. I think I did okay, but again it was hard to really know for sure. It was going into my teenage years and beyond that I got off track.

I became a bit of a wild child. My parents tried to shelter me from everything. My mother didn't like it when I wanted to listen to Rock Music. They didn't want anything bad happening to me. So of course, I had to rebel. I went out. A lot. This was during my high school and college years. I really didn't take care of myself too well, but thankfully I did learn better.

When I was in my twenties, I actually put together a fundraising festival for JDF in Charleston, South Carolina. With my father being so involved in the organization I felt I had to contribute to my own cause. I found out that putting together an event like that was a huge task and I needed help. Lots of help. I enlisted the assistance of friends and family. At this time in my life, I was taking guitar lessons from a local "legend" at a music store. Because of him the owner of that store stepped up to help and got a local radio station involved. We had several bands play, we had t-shirts made, food and perfect weather. It was a great event but stressful. I was so stressed in the weeks before the event, especially when I realized that the paperwork needed to sell alcohol on site had not been filed. I was so passionate about what I was doing, that I actually quit my job on the spot to drive to Columbia. It was the fastest I had ever driven and I made it just in time. It was quite a learning experience, and one that would serve me well later.

Again, I did not always make the best choices. I sometimes would hang out with the wrong people, or date the wrong people. I ate things I shouldn't, drank more than I should have and sometimes I may have even forgotten to take my insulin on schedule. I made mistakes but I don't beat myself up over them. Everything that I did in the past brought me to where I am today, so I wouldn't change a thing.

Before going into high school, I was a model student. Got good grades, was always the most attentive and polite and tried my best to never do anything wrong. When I got to high school, I was in the Advanced Placement classes, which was new for the school. I think that I was a bit overwhelmed with all of it. I went from an 8th grade class of just 11 students to the high school which was well over 200. I was trying to adjust to that, to the advanced classes and to being a teenager with diabetes. I also wanted to fit in. I know that most teenagers act out and rebel, so I was no different in that aspect. However, looking back I know that I should have been more careful and more observant. I was putting my health at risk by being rebellious and I am very very lucky to have no complications because of my teens and 20's.

I did not have the typical college experience. I chose to attend the College of Charleston which was about a 20-minute drive from my house. I did not stay on campus, I lived at home. I also had a part time job. I also went out with friends. All of these "excuses" kept me from doing well in college and I ended up dropping out I believe it was the beginning of my junior year. Not to mention that I changed my major a few times so the courses I needed kept changing. I wish I would have been more diligent and actually graduated. That is my one regret in life.

All in all, I did okay with my health during all of this, or at least I believe I did. Like I said, there were no glucometers available then for testing at home. I just took my insulin twice a day without really knowing what my blood sugar levels really were. I just did it because that is what I was supposed to do. I was simply taking my "prescribed" dosage from my doctor. I didn't know to do anything else but follow doctor's orders. Knowing what I know now, I can't believe that I am still alive. I could have had a really high blood sugar number and that prescribed dosage wouldn't be enough. Or, I could have had a low number and the prescribed dosage could cause insulin shock, seizure, or worse.

How to help your teen deal with a chronic disease

If I were to go back and talk to my 12-year-old self about Type 1 or give my parents advice about helping me cope with my diagnosis, here is the approach I would take:

Actionable steps to take:

1. **Find a diabetes educator AND a support group.** At the very least, find someone to talk to about the diagnosis. Having a support system in place is so vital to managing the disease, staying positive and for dealing with daily struggles.

2. **Do your own research on dietary changes.** Look up ways to cook healthier meals. One great idea is for parents and teens to take a cooking class together.

3. **Test your blood sugar levels often.** That is the only way to know how you are doing, whether your medication is working or not working, and how you are responding to food, stress and more. Make sure to keep records of your testing.

4. **An even better way of monitoring blood sugar levels is to get a CGM or continuous glucose monitor.** This is a device worn on the body with a sensor that goes just

underneath the skin. It constantly measures glucose levels and the sensor is changed every 10 days. This takes away the need for finger sticks and can really improve control.

5. **Talk to the doctor.** Share blood sugar logs and ask questions. You need to be involved in your own health care. You know how you are feeling much better than the doctor and together, you can make a great team in improving your health and diabetes management.

I have added a few resources at the back of this book that may be of help to you or your teen diagnosed with diabetes. The biggest thing to remember is that this is your health journey. It will take time and effort, but with consistency, you and your teen can figure out together what will work.

CHAPTER 2:
MY HOLISTIC HEALTH EXPERIMENT

After almost 20 years of just "surviving" with diabetes, I decided it was time to really live and thrive. That was my new intention. I remembered my next door neighbor and was reminded that I needed to do better. It was time for some major changes.

I followed a man to Myrtle Beach where I tried several jobs until I found the perfect place. It was a veterinary hospital. I loved it there. I loved the people and I loved all of the animals. It was a second home to me. Eventually the man left, and I stayed. I had rented a small house in a small town about 20 minutes from work and I went back to school to try to finish my degree. This led me to the man who later became my husband. I always tell people that I moved to Myrtle Beach for the wrong reasons, but I stayed for the right ones. I am so glad I did.

A few months after moving, I found a job with a veterinary hospital. I was hired as front desk staff. I loved it there, especially the animals. I became very attached to many. I soon worked in every area of the hospital including assisting in surgeries and even working in the kennels. I was constantly busy, rarely stopping to check my blood sugar. By this time of course, I had a glucometer so I could check to see exactly what my blood sugar levels were. But sadly, I reverted back to old habits of just "doing what I was told," taking my insulin as prescribed and testing myself maybe once or twice a day, depending on the day.

This is not a good way to do things, as we know. I remember several occasions where I would have mini seizures while working. I would go so low that I would have a hard time speaking or knowing what I was even saying. One day in particular, I was holding a puppy that had come in for an appointment. I had to take him back into the hospital for a few tests and then I just held onto him and walking around aimlessly. I am certain the owners were worried when I didn't return to the exam room in a reasonable amount of time. One of my coworkers recognized that something was wrong and got some orange juice for me out of the break room refrigerator and she took the puppy back into the room for me and finished the appointment. I was embarrassed and a little scared once I was coherent again.

I stayed at the veterinary hospital for close to 18 years and I still consider the doctors and staff there like family. But I realized that I had other aspirations and other things to do and that it was time to move on.

After leaving the vet hospital, my boyfriend and my father helped me purchase a small health food store in the small town of Conway, SC. I knew nothing about running a business. I knew very little about health food, but I was trying to be healthy again and my boyfriend was a chiropractor so I thought I would give it a shot. It was a lovely little store. There were a few rows of shelves with different food items, supplements, bulk grains and spices and even a small café in the back. I started serving lunches daily. I added a couple of couches to the shop and it became a reading area so people could enjoy their fresh juice, coffee or lunch and read. I learned so very much during my time there. I kept a copy of Prescription for Nutritional Healing by my side at all times, along with a highlighter. People came in asking questions and if I didn't know the answer I looked it up immediately. It was the hardest I had ever worked in my life. Again, I really knew nothing about running a business and very little about finances. I would give people advice on different foods and supplements and they would take that information and buy a cheaper product at Walmart. I had several of those people come in later and actually TELL me that my prices were too high so they purchased products that I had recommended in another store. I felt very frustrated and angry. Quite frankly I felt used. I spent time with them and tried to help them as much as I could and they opted to support a big box store instead of the person that pointed them in the right direction. I did continue to offer help to customers and I had some loyal people who came in weekly. I did the best I could.

While owning the shop, I started developing psoriasis all over my body. I had never had it before, didn't know much about it. I knew that I was working very hard every day and constantly stressed. I thought that maybe that was a trigger. I had it on my legs, arms, scalp, everywhere. It was embarrassing and I covered up all of the time. I tried cream after cream. Out of desperation, I went to a dermatologist who put me on the prescription Enbrel. I took a few doses. It was an injection, but I was used to giving myself injections so that wasn't the problem. The problem was the list of possible side effects that included death. I decided that it wasn't worth the risk so I stopped. I then started researching possible ways to treat my skin naturally.

I still had many books on natural healing from the shop and by now, the internet had become my best friend. I found a lot of information about detoxing and how many toxins the colon holds onto. So I bit the bullet and scheduled a colonic. I actually used to help give some animals in the veterinary hospital colonics so I was really not looking forward to it. To say it was an uncomfortable experience would be a tremendous understatement. Not to mention embarrassing. However, about a week after the first treatment, I noticed improvement in my skin. It had helped! We decided to test our water for chemicals. That was another idea I got from the fabulous internet. The level of chlorine coming from the tap was high for swimming pool standards. We purchased a shower filter and I noticed even more improvement. After 3 colonics, my skin was clear. So we upgraded to a whole house filtration system and I didn't have any more skin problems, except for once a year one spot would pop up when it was time to flush the system. Then it would go away. I treated myself naturally and it worked—without the risk of death. Owning the health food store and reading those books on a daily basis, really taught me the value of natural medicine, natural treatments and healthy living. After my skin was clear, I was absolutely a believer!

After closing the shop, I needed something to do. I needed a job. Having the shop engrained a new belief system and purpose in me, so I did not necessarily want to go back to the veterinary hospital. I wanted to help people with their health by more natural means. My boyfriend and I started a new business venture with help from another chiropractor friend. We set up a kiosk in one of the local malls and I did spinal screenings on shoppers. I would then refer them to one of our participating doctors that was nearest to them. That job was all about educating people. Educating them on the spine, the nervous system and what chiropractic is. I had a lot of downtime and I got many comments about "quackery" but all in all, I think we helped a lot of people. I had a few people come back to the kiosk thanking me for sending them to the chiropractor. The mall was close to The House of Blues in Myrtle Beach so we often had bands coming through the mall and they would stop out of curiosity. A few times we actually got some backstage passes to shows because we helped them so much. That was a big bonus!

While running the kiosk I knew that I wanted to make a bigger impact, make a bigger difference in the community. I saw so many unhealthy, unhappy and overweight people everyday. I could see it on their faces, in the way they walked, in their body language. It hurt to see people in so much pain and so unhealthy. I wanted to change that. I knew from all of the studying that I had done with the health food store as well as what my mother taught me about researching and questioning things, that perhaps I could make a difference. Maybe, just maybe I could help improve the health of others, the way I was improving my own health. The health food store was great, but it only reached a very small population. I needed to do something on a bigger scale.

I went back for another visit with my best friend, the internet. I looked for ways to "spread the message" on natural health. I could build a website. I could write a book. I could become a speaker. That was definitely out because I did NOT like speaking in front of people. Every time I did, my face would turn a million shades of red. Then I saw that there were natural health expos all over the country, just not in my area. So I decided that I could do that. I already had experience putting together an event, so I started by contacting the local convention center and finding out what dates were available. I reserved one of the exhibit halls and then started contacting potential vendors. I didn't do any market research or surveys about what people wanted to see. I just did it. We had a two-day event and about 30 vendors total, maybe more. I even brought in a guest speaker, a veterinarian that taught at the chiropractic college where my boyfriend attended. He spoke about chiropractic help for pets and people loved it. This was in 2003. We did not make any money on the venture, we actually lost due to the high expense of the convention center, the table and chair rentals and the insurance, but we started something for sure. This event went on for 4 more years, never really making any money, but making some progress. In 2006, with the help of one of our past vendors, we formed our "no profit" company into a nonprofit organization called The Wellness Council for South Carolina.

While running the health food store and healing myself of psoriasis, I also gained a good bit of weight, 20-30 pounds to be exact. I was living with my boyfriend and followed his lead on eating. I ate what he ate. I exercised, but not nearly enough. I also got sick a good bit. After the shop closed and we started the Spinal Assessment Center, I also went back to work at the Veterinary Hospital. I would take a few months off every year while putting the Wellness Expo together. I was stressed, sick and overweight, and scattered. In 2005, the most amazing thing happened. While in Las Vegas for a chiropractic conference, he proposed to me, on top of the Eiffel Tower! I was speechless and started crying after I said yes. We had an audience for the occasion and everyone applauded. We then walked from Paris to New York (Vegas style) and had dinner with family.

It was soon after that I decided to take control of my health again. I had been receiving newsletters via email from Dr. Joseph Mercola. He is an Osteopath with an office in Chicago. I decided to make an appointment to see him. I set off on my first trip to the Windy City. While there, I did happen to notice a David's Bridal nearby so I took a cab and tried on dresses by myself. It wasn't much fun, but it was something to do. I had multiple appointments with the doctor on staff at the clinic and many tests done. Blood tests, applied kinesiology, and more. They were trying to determine underlying causes of illness. I went home after being told that I had a gluten allergy. I was given a list of foods to cut out of my diet. I did this immediately, without looking back. Without even trying, I lost 20 pounds. The colds were much less frequent, almost non-existent. I felt lighter and happier. Some foods I added back in but I have never once added the gluten back.

I slimmed down quite a bit for the wedding and my skin was clear. We got married in 2006, the same year we started the nonprofit. In that same year, my husband also purchased a new building for his office, renovated it and moved in, all in the same month as the wedding. We like to do as much as possible in a short amount of time. A few months later was another Wellness Expo. It was a crazy, stressful, and extremely exciting time.

Recommendations for starting with holistic health

Actionable steps to take:

1. **Again, do your research.** If you are given a prescription by your doctor, ask questions, look up the medication online, and find out what the possible side effects are.

2. **Look up alternative methods of treatment.**

3. **If possible, find a naturopath or functional medicine practitioner** to work together with your current doctor. If everybody works together, the outcomes are generally much better.

4. **Start a journal.** Keep track of things that you do, eat, drink, and any medications or supplements you take. This way if you have a reaction, you can go back to your journal to see what may be the cause. Review this journal regularly and pay attention to how you feel. Journaling is a great way to get in touch with your own body, so you can actively participate in the healing process. This can help with all areas of health.

Checklist for figuring out if holistic health is right for you:

- Are you taking a lot of medications, but still having problems?

- Do you dislike some of the side effects you experience when taking your medication?

- Are you tired all of the time? Do you feel depressed?

- Do you want to work towards being truly well and not just free from sickness? Keep in mind that being healthy is more than just the absence of disease.

- While we can't believe everything that is on the Internet, it is still a great place to get loads of information on anything and everything. The more you research and the more information you gather, the better and more informed decisions you can make about your own health.

Chapter 3:
Accidental Advocate in the Hospital

In 2008, I became pregnant. A little girl. We were so excited! Everyone was. We decided we wanted a natural, home birth. We hired both a doula and a midwife to assist. We took classes. I did everything I was supposed to do. It was the healthiest I had ever been. My doctor was so thrilled at every appointment because I was doing so well and my blood sugar was perfect. We got the nursery ready and it was perfect as well. It had a zoo theme and it was beautiful. My family threw me a surprise baby shower. It was wonderful. I went for my 36-week appointment and was told I was in the beginning of labor. A few days before the appointment, my water broke. That was a Friday. At least I am pretty sure that is what happened. But I wasn't in labor. I was told that sometimes the baby could accidentally cause the water to break before it was actually time. I took great care to keep everything clean and sanitized. The following Tuesday, I had a high fever and went directly to the emergency room. I never saw the doctor. Not once. It was late so the nurses did the exam. I was sent home and told to take some Tylenol PM and drink plenty of water. The next night I felt like I was in labor so we called the doula and midwife. I walked around the house, pacing, breathing and drinking water. I laid in a warm tub of water. Things were not quite ready to happen. On Friday, I had my regular checkup. My mother in law drove me since I couldn't sit quite right. They told me I was in labor then.

They went to check the heartbeat. That was when things went completely wrong. There was no heartbeat. Nothing. Silence. I was taken to the hospital immediately.

Everything was a blur. To be honest, I don't remember a lot after that. I called my husband and told him what was going on and did what I needed to, but I was in a deep deep fog. They gave me an epidural, which previously I had decided against for delivery, but at that point I could care less about anything. I couldn't feel anything. I was in absolute shock and completely numb. She was gone before we could even meet her. I delivered her the next morning, or so I am told. Again, I don't remember much about days or times. We were able to hold Hanna once. That was her name. Hanna. Hanna Tegan Falk. We held her just once. I wish I could have frozen that moment in time.

I stayed in that hospital for two weeks. My fever was stubborn and it was a fever of unknown origin. They pumped my body with every antibiotic they had in stock. Nothing worked. They told me they wanted to do exploratory surgery and most likely remove my uterus. I told them I would walk myself right out of the hospital before I would let that happen. Their response to that was that I would be leaving "Against Medical Advice" and that insurance would not pay for anything then. So I asked to be transferred elsewhere. So they begrudgingly sent me to The Medical University of South Carolina, two-three hours away. I was sent in an ambulance. That was not a pleasant ride, a little bumpy and uncomfortable, although the paramedics were nice. Once I arrived, the doctors reviewed my chart and took me off of all medications. All of the antibiotics. Miraculously, my fever went away. Because I rarely take any prescriptions, other than my insulin, my body was having a reaction to the onslaught of medications. Whatever infection that was there to begin with had been long gone. Just imagine if I had stayed in the other hospital. Exploratory surgery and hysterectomy.

One thing I noticed at both hospitals was the food. Hospital food is never good, but it's even worse when you have a gluten allergy. Did I mention that? When I was close to home, I had family that could bring me food. At MUSC, I had to rely mostly on their menu. And for a teaching hospital, they knew absolutely nothing about a gluten allergy, or gluten itself. I had to work with the food manager and review the entire menu. I had to physically point out what I could and could not have. They had no clue. I was appalled.

I finally was able to leave MUSC and go home after about a week. I was thankful for that, but uncertain what to do next. We had prepared for so long for our daughter's arrival, and I went home empty-handed and just, empty.

I was still physically recovering from everything and emotionally trying to recover, neither of which was easy. Of course the physical recovery couldn't come close to the emotional. Every day, I would sit in the rocking chair in the nursery, and cry. I would look at the clothes and toys. Every day I went over everything in my head. I blamed everyone and everything, but mostly I blamed myself for not knowing that something was wrong. It was the worst thing I could ever think of going through and something that I never imagined in my worst nightmare, but there I was. I think I pushed people, including my husband, away because he reminded me of everything we had lost. I regret that every day.

I finally was able to pick myself up, dust myself off and move forward. I was starting to get pretty good at that. I thought back about my time in the local hospital and how much I had to stand up for myself and say no to very radical treatments. I had to say no to what they wanted to do, since they didn't even know what they would be looking for. Exploratory surgery are really two words that should never go together. Any type of surgery, routine or not, can be dangerous and the doctor should really know what to look for, remove or repair before going in. I had to be my own advocate.

That Christmas, my in-laws bought us a copy of the workout P90X. I had heard of it but really wasn't sure what it was all about. We finally opened it in January. Every morning, 6 days a week, we woke up at 6am 0 and did the video for the day. Most lasted about and hour, the yoga was an hour and a half. We took our before photos and planned on completing the 90-day program. After about a month and half in, I started having trouble breathing. I would have to stop repeatedly to catch my breath. I think my husband just thought I was faking it at first, but I was struggling a little more each and every day. I finally talked my husband into taking an x-ray of my lungs. It showed some definite damage to my lung tissue. My lungs were white and mottled when they should be dark and clear. But we still didn't know what I had. After a couple of months, I went to an Integrative Doctor to get checked out. She did blood work on me and other tests. She did some Vitamin C chelation therapy on me, which was done with an IV, along with other treatments. Before getting any diagnosis, she gave me an injection of Vitamin D, which does help with your immune system.

The bloodwork came back and showed that I had high calcium levels so she sent me to get a bone scan done. I walked into that office with the order from the doctor and the reason listed for my visit (my diagnosis) was lung cancer. I was not aware of this diagnosis but the woman working at the imaging center happened to be a friend and she almost fell over upon reading that.

I had the scan done and I went home and awaited the results. It was a long, agonizing wait. When I finally had the results faxed to me, it took me a long time before I could bring myself to even look at the piece of paper. I was terrified. What else was I going to have to go through? Hadn't I gone through enough already?

I mustered up the courage and pulled the paper from the fax machine and started reading. No cancer detected. None. I did not have cancer. The other possible diagnosis, and the most likely was something called Sarcoidosis. I had absolutely no idea what that was, so the internet was once again my best friend.

I started reading everything I could find on sarcoidosis. What it was, what causes it, what happens, treatments, natural treatments...anything and everything I could get my hands on. I found out that one of the signs of sarcoidosis, besides the shortness of breath and wheezing, was having red rashes or lumps on the skin. I had previously noticed these but was told by the dermatologist that I went to that they were just pimples and not to worry. So, I went to my general practitioner and asked to have a skin biopsy done. This biopsy confirmed my sarcoidosis diagnosis. I was amazed that after everything, I had to be the one to ask for the test which gave me my official diagnosis. The doctors that I saw, either didn't see a problem or just tried to medicate me the way they did every other breathing or skin issue that they saw. I had to do the research and ask for the test. Again, I had to stand up for myself and be my own advocate. This was something else I was getting pretty good at.

So, I had a name for what was making me sick. Now what? I first did some more reading on the disease and saw that Vitamin D, while it helps most people, actually makes sarcoidosis worse. It causes the granulomas that exist in my lungs to replicate faster. So that injection given to me previously likely did more harm than good. Again, treating without a true diagnosis.

Through more reading, I learned of some patients who were helped by a specific antibiotic with long term treatment. I gave this information to my general practitioner who looked it up and wrote a prescription. She also referred me to a local pulmonologist. I scheduled that appointment and did the required x-rays and breathing tests. He told me what I already knew, that my lungs were damaged and there were granulomas everywhere. He prescribed prednisone, which is the standard course of treatment. He could not tell me what the cause of sarcoidosis was. He really could not tell me much about it at all other than the fact that it could affect other parts of my body, which I already knew from my own research. I told him that I was diabetic so prednisone would be a problem, but he assured me that it was what I needed. I went home and did as I was told.

Day 1 of the prednisone did not sit well with me. Steroids and diabetes do not mix well. My blood sugar skyrocketed. My breathing was greatly improved and I was able to get back on my elliptical machine with no problems. However, I could not eat much due to the blood sugar issues. I couldn't sleep much either because the medicine made me jittery and a little hyper. Plus, I was up every couple of hours checking my glucose levels and taking insulin as needed to lower it. I was also very cranky. Nobody wanted to be around me. Even with all of the problems, I finished the prescription. I learned however, that even though I knew how to handle it, I didn't want to ever take that medicine again.

I maintained pretty well for awhile after that, but still had problems with shortness of breath, wheezing and difficulty walking long distances. If we went of our town, whether on vacation or to a conference, I always felt like I was holding everyone back. I couldn't keep up. I couldn't walk like everyone else could, and certainly not at the same pace. I felt broken.

Again, I started more research online about natural treatments because I couldn't take prescriptions long term, and quite frankly didn't want to. I found all types of "miracle cures" online. They all promised to be THE answer. Some were diets, some were pills. Some involved way too much time and sacrifice to ever be sustainable for me. Others promised relief as long as you purchased a book or subscribed to their website. I am usually willing to try anything if I think it could help, but some of it was just too much. There is a lot of that on the internet. Too many "miracle cures".

I came across something called Soup A and Soup B from a company called Wei Laboratories. They only sell through doctors' offices. By doctors, I mean holistic doctors. Wei Laboratories is a Chinese herbal company. Since my husband was a chiropractor, I did a health evaluation form with them and worked with them and got the soup products. I started them right away. These soups are not something you had for lunch or dinner. They are rather, liquid supplements that you take three times a day, along with a couple of other products they recommend. The soups came in big glass jars, like a mason jar, and looked (and tasted) like mud. But I took them every day. I can honestly say that they helped—a great deal in fact.

I noticed a difference after about a week and a half. I had more energy, I could breathe better and my endurance was much improved. I was so happy! I told my husband that I felt like I had my life back.

Every time I received a Soup shipment, it was like Christmas morning, but instead of toys, I got jars filled with liquid that tasted like dirt. But I loved it! It was helping.

I must have done the Soup protocol for 6-8 months. I was doing so well. Things were looking up.

In January 2013, e were set to go to the Parker Seminar in Las Vegas. Parker is the Chiropractic school that my husband attended and their seminars are the biggest and best, bringing doctors from all over the world, guest speakers and more. I was so excited. I always left these seminars inspired, hopeful and ready to change the world!

The seminar was held in one of the large casinos on the strip, since over 1,000 doctors were in attendance. In order to get to the classes and the expo to visit with vendors, you had to walk through the casino—the smoke-filled casino. No matter what time of day or night, people smoked nonstop. Even to go to the hotel gym, you had to walk through the smoke. We were only there for a few days, so I just dealt with it. I wasn't going to be the party pooper. I wanted to have fun like everyone else. So we enjoyed the seminar, met some great people and learned a lot. A few weeks after returning home, my health started in a downward spiral. My breathing got significantly worse. I blamed it on all of the cigarette smoke I had to deal with on the trip.

The months went by and I continued to get worse. I was teaching an after school program at a local middle school once a week at this time. My focus was on nutrition and exercise, yet I could really do no exercise. Some of the kids had to help me bring in my supplies every week because I was just unable to do it. I was trying to teach them about being healthy, while I myself was unhealthy. I felt like such a fraud. But I kept moving forward. I did what I had to do.

That August, we went on vacation to Aruba. Again, I had to walk slowly. I was again slowing everyone down. But I still was able to relax and enjoy myself. I had to look on the bright side. Otherwise, I would just cry all of the time and feel sorry for myself. I have to admit; I have done that sometimes. More often than I would really like to say.

In November of 2013, we had the opportunity to take yet another trip to Seattle to another chiropractic conference. We had never been and had really been looking forward to seeing the sights. It was a rough trip though.

On the flight over, we had two layovers. I remember having a really hard time going from gate to gate. Even just getting off the plane and into the terminal was a struggle. My husband had to actually get an airport wheelchair for me to get to our gate. It was on the other side of the airport and there was absolutely no way I would make it without assistance. It was extremely humiliating.

In the hotel it was no different. I could barely walk 10 feet without stopping to catch my breath. I had to be around my husband's peers and pretend like everything was fine. I dressed up and did what I could. We went out at night, ate and drank and had a great time. I was just really slow. Thankfully he tried to keep closer to my pace so I didn't get lost. We went through Pike's Market, saw the first Starbucks, had dinner at the top of the Space Needle, and saw everything we wanted to see in Seattle I believe. It's a beautiful city. One night we visited the EMP Museum, the Experience Music Project. That was quite a place! They had team building exercises where they went on a scavenger hunt through the museum. I stayed behind in the bar while this went on because I didn't want to slow down the team and be the reason they lost. After, we toured around a bit and was able to really experience the music industry. The teams all created their own music video, we played different instruments in soundproof rooms and I even got to sing with the band Heart. It was a recorded version of course, but I still was able to cross that off my bucket list. At the end of the night, we had to take the long way around to get out. I was having trouble and eventually he picked me up, put me on his back and carried me to the door. Again, it was humiliating, but fortunately nobody there seemed to notice.

At the conference, there was a doctor from Seattle set up at the expo, a Naturopath. My husband talked to her about my condition and called me downstairs to meet her. It was the end of the seminar and all of the vendors were packing up, but she stayed to talk with me. She talked to me about different things, how I was feeling, my breathing difficulties, explaining Chinese herbs and homeopathy to me and seemed to feel that she could indeed help me. She sold us a few items from her table on the spot. Two of these were topical creams; one for inflammation and one to help the other penetrate faster. The other product she sold us was a three-part detox kit. They were liquids that helped detox the liver, kidneys and lymphatic system. She was explaining how they worked but honestly all I heard was that it could help. We took the products back up to the room and I immediately applied some of the creams. I decided to wait on the detox until we returned home. This was a Saturday night. I actually felt a little better just from the topical creams. I walked a little bit farther than I had previously in the day. So I was good with that. I applied more before going to bed and the next morning before flying home.

We got home on Sunday and on Monday morning I started the detox, with the exact dosage of each liquid that she told me. Two days later, the change was dramatic. I could breathe! I could walk more. I could do things. I was unbelievably happy at this point. It only took 2 days for the improvement.

I worked with this naturopath for a couple of years, since she was helping me with multiple issues. I did end up going back to the soups since they really helped me the most.

There was a point where another pulmonologist that I saw told me I needed to be on oxygen 24/7 and that I needed to be on the transplant list. When he told me that, I walked out of his office and never went back. A week later, I was in Costa Rica hiking half a mile up a volcano. No oxygen tank. Granted, I was a little slow still, but I did it. My general practitioner has since proclaimed me a miracle. He has seen the before and after lung x-rays and the incredible difference in the two. It's actually quite dramatic as you can see.

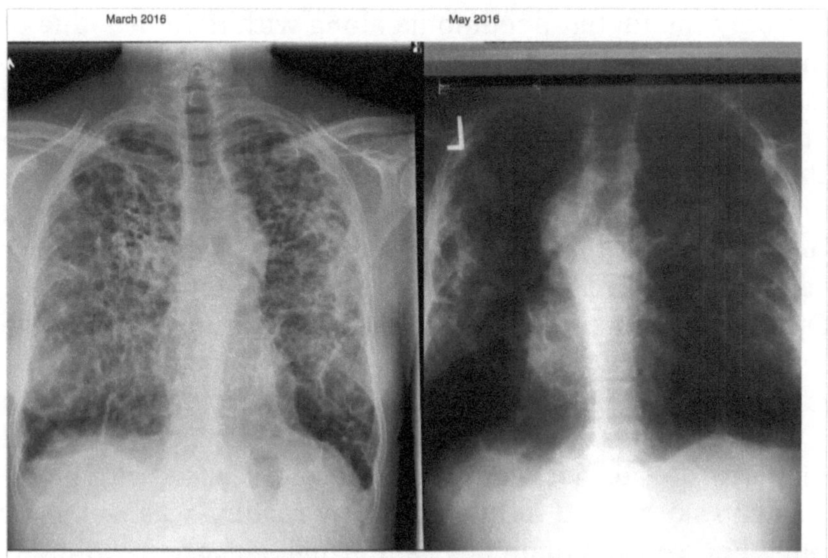

So yet again, I was doing my own research, being my own health advocate and really, educating the doctors a little each time I saw them.

That is why it is so important to do your own research. If a doctor wants me to take a medication, I immediately look it up to find out what it is, what it does, possible side effects as well as more natural, and safer alternatives. Unless it is an emergency situation, I usually decline the prescription. My doctors now know what I will and won't do. They see me results and no longer argue with me. In fact, sometimes they ask me questions. Remember that your doctor works for you, not the other way around. And the best way to deal with a health issue is to work together. If you don't like what they have to say, then get a second or even third opinion. It is your health. It's your body and you are your own best advocate!

While I was getting my lung health under control, I was still having some severe lows in blood sugar, so I went ahead and ordered the CGM device in December of 2017. It arrived in January, along with the flu. Unfortunately, I got not only the flu but pneumonia along with it. In fact, due to my previous difficulty with my lungs and sarcoidosis, I was having such a hard time breathing that I called 911 and had an ambulance pick me up from my home and drive me to the emergency room which was only about 3 miles away. I was put in the CCU (critical care unit) and was on a breathing tube for I believe 5 or 6 days. I honestly don't remember a lot. I was in the hospital for a total of 11 days. During that time, they really had no idea how to manage type 1 diabetes. Because I was having difficulty with my lungs, they gave me steroids to help open up my airways so I could breathe. That is standard. However, steroids and diabetes do not get along. The steroids caused my blood sugar to sky rocket! At one point, my reading was well over 600. For those unfamiliar, a normal glucose reading is around 100. So that 600+ reading was dangerously high and was doing some serious organ damage. My husband demanded that they lower it with insulin. They argued saying that it is standard protocol to lower it slowly. Knowing that the longer it stayed that elevated, the more damage it was doing, he argued more and eventually they listened.

A few days later, I was finally taken off the ventilator. For the next day or two I was put on a "liquid diet" only due to the irritation of the breathing tube. Plus, they wanted to make sure I didn't choke. I will tell you, that as a diabetic with a gluten allergy this liquid diet did not work well. My husband told them about the gluten allergy. I told them every time they brought any form of what they called "food" yet it was not written in my records anywhere! For breakfast they would bring me flavorless grits, fruit juice and yogurt. I argued that scrambled eggs would be just as easy to swallow and more easily digested but they were not allowed to go against protocol. For lunch and dinner, I always got boxed mashed potatoes with some kind of gravy that I am sure had flour in it. I kept arguing and finally they listened. They wrote GLUTEN ALLERGY on my chart and I got some halfway decent food that I could eat.

I was finally moved out of CCU and into a regular room that was about half the size of the other room. (I think my clothes closet at home is actually bigger.) One night they brought me dinner. It was a big plate of pasta (gluten free) with spaghetti sauce. Then they checked my blood sugar. Had I been at home, I would always check myself before dinner and give an insulin injection at least 30 minutes prior to eating, more if it was high. This particular time it was over 200. I said "ok, I need to get my insulin now". The nurse said "no, you had an injection a few hours ago. You need to go ahead and eat. You aren't scheduled for another dose for 2 hours." Obviously that earlier injection didn't work and I needed more. She said that she could not give me any insulin unless the doctor ok'd it. I told her that I did in fact know what I was talking about as a person who had been dealing with diabetes for well over 30 years and was also a diabetes educator. The nurse then gave me the "eye roll" before calling the doctor. He of course, gave the ok and I got my insulin injection. My blood sugar came down and I was eventually able to eat my now cold pasta. If I had just let things be and not demand the insulin my blood sugar would probably have spiked to 600 again. I knew what all of those carbohydrates would do. Why didn't they? I still can't understand why they would test and not treat at the same time, especially if it was elevated. If it had been low, they would have rushed in and made me drink a few cups of juice. But high blood sugar did not seem to concern them much even though it could cause serious complication and permanent organ damage if left untreated. They just didn't seem to get it. It still baffles me. The hospitals, doctors, nurses are great when it comes to emergency medicine and situations but there is a lot lacking when it comes to caring for those with chronic conditions.

When I was finally given a clean bill of health and told that I could go home, they still had me on oxygen. I had to ask for a portable tank in case I needed to go to any appointments while I was recovering and needed a little bit of help with my breathing. I had to ask for it.

So after all of that, once I got home I was able to get myself back on track, get my lungs strong again, (using the Soups that I had used before) and started to feel normal.

I thought about everything that went on in the hospital and I started working on a new project; writing new hospital protocol for treating patients with diabetes. This is a project that I am currently still working on. My own doctor is on board to help me with it and get it into the right hands. It seems to be a daunting task but one that I really care deeply about and it is definitely needed. A protocol written from a diabetic's point of view and own experience could really help others and possibly save lives. I won't give up.

Recommendations for being a health advocate for yourself or others in the hospital

Actionable steps to take:

1. **Speak up.** You have to say something if you know something is wrong or if doctors and nurses are not listening to you. Keep saying what you think over and over until they listen and acknowledge your concerns. You deserve an explanation for whatever is happening to your body!

2. **Write things down.** Make sure to keep a record of everything going on, if you are able, of course. If you cannot take notes for yourself, find someone you trust to keep track of what's happening. Even the strongest advocates need help sometimes.

3. **Have some support in place.** Enlist the support of a spouse, family member, or close friend. Have someone there with you who knows what is going on and can also be an advocate if you are incapacitated. It also can be helpful to talk through health decisions with others who are absolutely on your side.

4. **Remember that doctors, nurses, and the hospital staff work FOR YOU.** They may have a lot of initials after their names, but you are the expert when it comes to your own body and they need to listen to you. Don't be afraid and don't back down. Now is not the time to be shy. Your health could be at stake.

CHAPTER 4:
PUBLIC ADVOCATE RUNNING A NON-PROFIT

Everything to this point has been about having a problem that, according to my MD's, could not be solved naturally. I honestly loved being able to prove them wrong. But underneath it all, I was still a diabetic with a pancreas that did not do its job.

I have been very diligent about my blood sugars for at least the last 10-12 years. Like I said, my teenage years and early 20's were completely different, but I learned from my mistakes and I changed. It did help when the at-home glucometers became available and relatively inexpensive so that all I had to do to find out my blood sugar number was prick my finger, put a tiny drop of blood on a test strip and 10 seconds later, I could make decisions on food or insulin based on where I was.

The nonprofit organization that we started in 2006 actually started out as The Wellness Council for Coastal South Carolina, a small community nonprofit that wanted to educate and inspire people about better nutrition, health, physical fitness and environment. I was encouraged by a gentleman who had put together another similar nonprofit in North Carolina and he thought we could do well with it and reach more people than some of our previous ventures. We started out wanting to teach ANYONE and EVERYONE about better health. As Executive Director, I gave speeches, wrote articles, set up at health fairs and went to schools to teach kids. We even started an after-school program at a local middle school. The program was called Green S.P.A.R.K. (Shaping Potential and Reaching Kids) and its lessons included nutrition, cooking, exercise, recycled arts, renewable energy information as well as gardening. That program ran for four-five years and was so much fun. There were a few times, when working with certain kids, that the teachers and parents actually thanked me for turning the students around and helping them make healthier choices. Of course the program was short lived because of changes within the school and the after-school program choices. I am hopeful that one day we can start the program up again and reach more students in the future. In fact, we are in the process of bringing it back, but in our own facility rather than inside the school system. We are optimistic that we can make it work and help the kids the way we have done in the past.

For ten years, we tried to teach anyone and everyone about good nutrition, physical fitness and environment. I will tell you from experience that people really don't want to be told to eat their vegetables or drink more water. They hear it all the time. The see it on social media, on the news and inherently they know that is what they are supposed to do. But, change is hard. It takes work. Some people have to hit rock bottom before they will make any changes to their diet and their lifestyle. Even then, it can be a hard sell. But I am very stubborn and I keep trying. However, after ten years of doing the same things, we decided it was time to change things up a bit. It was time to go back to my roots.

In 2016, the state of South Carolina was ranked 6th highest in the country for people diagnosed with Type 2 diabetes. A whopping 13% of the population in South Carolina has diabetes. Type 2 is different from the Type 1 that I have. Most cases of Type 2 can be related to obesity, diet and lifestyle. In most cases, it can be greatly helped and even reversed with healthier choices and weight loss. Since I have been dealing with my own diabetes for most of my life, it seemed logical to use my experience and expertise to help others. At that point, I had my own diabetes under really good control and even my own doctor thought that I should teach others. So, we changed everything.

The organization went through a complete overhaul and rebranding. Our mission changed from educating "improving the health and wellness of the community at large as well as the environment,' to simply "educating those affected by diabetes." Both missions used nutrition education and physical activity education as a means of wellness, but now we target a specific audience. Since the diabetic population in our state was at such a high level with more that were likely undiagnosed, we felt that that direction would be the way to go and have the greatest impact. Again, people were tired of hearing about eating healthier and exercising more, but when it was about better diabetes management, it got their attention.

I gave my first diabetes workshop/presentation at my husband's chiropractic office to an audience of six people, five of whom were dealing with diabetes and one who was hoping to help her husband with his. It was close to a two-hour presentation with a good bit of discussion and question/answer. After the presentation was over, they all thanked me for the information I shared. One of the attendees even signed up for personal coaching with me, so I was pleased.

The following months, it became increasingly difficult to get people to attend the workshops. My doctor was even prescribing the workshops to his other diabetic patients because he knew it would help. So I changed things up a bit and started doing workshops that involved food. People love food and learning how to cook new things. So I did low carb cooking demos and tastings along with some of the information from the other presentations. It was a great deal more work but it was fun and rewarding. A couple of the attendees of these workshops improved their blood sugar control a great deal and that made me very happy. It felt good to actually be helping people.

Now let me backup a little bit. A few months prior to the rebranding and mission changes, I was in a car accident. I totaled my car. It happened because my blood sugar got way too low. I honestly didn't even know how I got to where the accident happened. I was in a dreamlike state and I can't even begin to tell you how much that scared me. I was physically okay thanks to my husband who adjusted me after the accident to help with any whiplash and other accident related injuries. But mentally, I was a basket case for awhile. I was terrified that I had hurt someone else and because of the simple fact of how and why the accident happened in the first place. It was really scary to not remember what you were doing when driving a vehicle, especially over a bridge. I am thankful that it wasn't as bad as it could have been. I believe someone was watching over me. Needless to say, I didn't drive for a little while and I had to get a new car. This is actually when I started looking into getting a CGM (continuous glucose monitor) that could tell me what my blood sugar levels were and which direction they were headed.

Back to the low carb workshops. Anything involving food usually brings the people. This was no different. I had people who attended every workshop. They were getting to taste the low carbs foods I prepared, take home recipes and were following the dietary recommendations. (I have a few recipes at the end of the book that are yummy and low carb!) I received some of the greatest testimonials from one woman in particular who was able to decrease her A1C (her level of control from the previous 3 months) and her doctor was very happy. She said she learned tips and information that she had never gotten from anyone else.

These workshops were a lot of fun but a lot of work and most of the time involved way more expense than I anticipated or got back. I ended up losing more money than I brought in so it really wasn't sustainable.

Recommendations for starting your own non-profit or supporting a local non-profit

Actionable steps to take:

1. **Do some research and see what is already being done that is similar to your passion.** If there is not already a local organization that does what you want to do, then you can move forward.

2. **Gather a list of interested parties, community leaders, friends and others** who have a similar interest and passion, to brainstorm ideas on mission, focus, goals as well as a name for the organization.

3. **It's best to get the help of an attorney** to do the necessary paperwork to apply for the nonprofit status.

4. **File the paperwork and wait.** This can take a few months up to a few years, so don't get discouraged.

5. **Don't give up and just keep moving forward.** The key to success is persistence and consistency.

CHAPTER 5:
LIFE IS A MARATHON

Like any business, a nonprofit organization must adjust, adapt and evolve. We changed our name to The Diabetes Wellness Council in 2018. We changed our website and logo again, our business cards, all our brochures, and basically everything. With these changes came some changes in me. Actually, it was probably the changes in me, all of my past experiences and my way of thinking that led to the big changes in the organization.

I thought back to the days when my husband and I would attend the big chiropractic conferences in Las Vegas and I imagined being up on that speaker stage. I decided that if I really wanted something I had to work for it. I had recently re-joined Toastmasters to get past my public speaking jitters. I thought that it might help me improve my workshops.

In Toastmasters, your first speech is called your "Ice Breaker" and it is meant to really introduce who you are to the group. My ice breaker speech was about being a person with diabetes. Actually most of my speeches are about different aspects and experiences I have had in dealing with diabetes for so long. I always try to be a little informative and educational with my talks. Plus, I found that talking about it all and educating others about the issues I have dealt with, helped me both physically and mentally. I recommend Toastmasters to everyone. Not only can it help you get over those awful public speaking jitters, it can improve your communication skills and help you deal with your own issues. I find it very therapeutic. When you are able to communicate more effectively, it can improve your work life, home life, and even help you become your own health advocate. I went on from there to speaking at different events across the country in front of hundreds of people. And to think back about how terrified I was about speaking in public, I knew that joining the group was the right decision.

In order to grow even more, I decided to take improv classes. That's right—improv. When most people think of improv they think of comedy, but it's really about being comfortable with who you are, being yourself, gaining confidence and not being afraid to fail. It's those times when we aren't afraid of failure or imperfection that we really grow. We take chances, we become more creative and become more of who we are meant to be. I can't even begin to tell you how much these two groups changed and improved my life.

I am more confident than ever. I am now traveling and speaking to different groups across the country. I am always still a little nervous, but nothing like I was before. Now I am confident in the knowledge that I have and its value. I never felt that way before, but because I am constantly learning, trying new things and growing, I can say that I have no doubts about what I am doing with my life.

I am a diabetic warrior. I am a chronic disease survivor. I am constantly growing and changing; constantly learning. Most importantly. I am my own health advocate. That is what everyone should be.

Recommendations for living with a chronic disease long term

Actionable steps to take:

1. Research, research, research.

2. Question everything.

3. Don't give up.

4. Support your gut and I don't mean your intuition. I mean get your gut healthy with a really good probiotic. Many chronic conditions can start in the gut because that is where a large part of your immune system lives. This is especially important if you have been on antibiotics.

Checklist for becoming a diabetic warrior:

- Remember that you are not alone.

- Understand that it CAN be managed and you can live a normal, healthy life, even with diabetes.

- Acceptance is important. You can manage and do well with diabetes much more, if you accept the diagnosis and move forward. Denial can only makes things worse.

- Let others know. The more people you have in your life that know and understand the diagnosis, the more support you will have and the better you can manage.

- Educate others.

- Research.

- Eat well, drink water, exercise and get enough rest. That is vital for any and all illness. Words to live by!

RESOURCES

The Diabetes Wellness Council:
https://diabeteswellnesscouncil.org

Juvenile Diabetes Research Foundation:
https://www.jdrf.org

American Diabetes Association:
Diabetes.org

For more information on Wei Laboratories:
WeiLab.com

Articles and information on natural health and healing:
Mercola.com

Toastmasters: Toastmasters.Org to find the chapter nearest you

Low Carb/Diabetic Friendly Recipes

Spaghetti Squash Casserole

1 large spaghetti squash

1 bag of frozen shrimp (or any protein you prefer)

1/2 cup sour cream

1/2 cup ricotta cheese

1/4 cup heavy cream

Parmesan cheese

Shredded cheese of your choice

Garlic powder (to taste)

Salt and pepper to taste

This is a very versatile recipe. You can use any protein source, or none. You can add spinach, mushrooms, broccoli, or any other vegetable of your choice.

Preheat oven to 350°. Cut squash in half lengthwise and remove seeds. Place upside down on plate or baking dish with some water. Cook in microwave on high for 10 minutes, or until soft. You can also cook in the stove. Scrape out the squash with a fork into bowl (be careful because it will be HOT!) Add seasoning, sour cream, ricotta, cornstarch mixture and heavy cream. Mix well and transfer to baking dish. Top with parmesan and shredded cheeses. Bake approximately 1 hour or until golden brown. It is best when made a day ahead of time.

Enjoy!

Chicken Parm

Traditional chicken parm recipes suggest frying the chicken. I don't eat a lot of fried foods, so I bake the chicken instead. I've altered this recipe slightly to fit my tastes.

4 skinless, boneless chicken breasts

1 jar your favorite pasta sauce (I love Rao's - Keto Approved)

Shredded mozzarella

Salt and pepper to taste

1/2 tsp garlic powder (or to taste)

1 tsp oregano

1/2 tsp basil

1/2 tsp parsley

Olive oil

Salt and pepper the chicken breasts and place in baking dish coated with olive oil. Preheat oven to 350°. Bake chicken until golden brown. Pour sauce over chicken, add seasonings, top with cheese and put back into the oven until sauce and cheese are bubbly.

Serve with pasta, risotto, potatoes or for a low carb meal, serve with mashed cauliflower.

Baked Tomatoes

I am all about using recipes that you can alter according to your tastes. I normally treat recipes as "guides" rather than "rule books." Feel free to make this recipe your own.

1 large beefsteak tomato

Seasoning of your choice

Cheese of your choice

The Ingredients of this recipe are completely up to you. It is very versatile. I love to add salt, pepper, garlic powder, and oregano for the seasoning.

Preheat oven to 350°. Slice tomato and put in greased baking dish. Sprinkle each slice with the seasoning of your choice and top with cheese. Bake in oven until cheese is melted and tomato slices are a little soft.

This makes a great side dish, especially in the spring and summer when the tomatoes are fresh from the garden.

Some of my favorite cheeses to use are feta, goat and mozzarella. If you use parmesan, you will not need any salt.

Cauliflower/Leek Soup

I love anything and everything cauliflower! Since I don't eat potatoes anymore, this was a great alternative to a soup I used to really love.

1 head cauliflower

1 leek bulb

1 garlic clove

Chicken broth

Olive oil

Salt and pepper to taste

Shredded cheese (optional)

Remove the stem from cauliflower and chop into large pieces. Thoroughly clean the leek bulb (leek bulbs can hold a lot of dirt, so double check.) Chop the leeks. Peel and chop the garlic. Place the vegetables and garlic in a pot with olive oil and sauté until leeks are soft. Add chicken broth until veggies are covered halfway and simmer until cauliflower is soft. Place contents into a food processor or blender and puree. Pour the blended mixture back into the pot and cook on low. Add salt and pepper to taste. Add more broth if necessary for the right consistency. If you like a thicker soup, add shredded cheese and stir.

Transfer to soup bowls and enjoy!

Oh My! Keto Chocolate Milk

4oz. unsweetened almond milk

4oz. heavy cream

1 tablespoon Chocolate MCT Oil Powder (I use Perfect Keto brand)

Liquid stevia to taste

Put the milk and cream in the glass, add the powder and stevia, blend and enjoy. (Tip: Add ice cubes to make a milkshake!)

Low Carb Shopping List

Some of the items I always keep on hand in the kitchen:

Avocadoes

Broccoli

Cucumbers

Spring mix for salads (or spinach)

Cauliflower

Eggplant

Zucchini (I LOVE zoodles (zucchini noodles))

Coconut Oil

Almond Flour

Coconut Flour

Himalayan Pink Salt

Swerve Sweetener (erythritol)

Liquid stevia (I use in my coffee and chocolate milk)

Heavy Whipping Cream

Eggs (I have my own hens so I am lucky to get really fresh eggs every day)

Kimchi (spicy, fermented cabbage - it's full of healthy probiotics)

Bone Broth (full of healthy collagen that is good for skin, hair, nails and more)

Chicken stock